Neuropathy Unveiled: Understanding and Managing Diabetic Nerve Damage

Copyright Page

TITLE: Neuropathy Unveiled: Understanding and Managing Diabetic Nerve Damage

1ST Edition

ISBN: 9798223342465

Table of Contents

Neuropathy Unveiled: Understanding and Managing Diabetic Nerve Damage 1

Chapter 1: Introduction to Neuropathy 2

Chapter 2: Diabetic Neuropathy..7

Chapter 3: Peripheral Neuropathy.. 13

Chapter 4: Autonomic Neuropathy 18

Chapter 5: Chemotherapy-induced Neuropathy........................ 23

Chapter 6: Small Fiber Neuropathy.. 28

Chapter 7: Idiopathic Neuropathy.. 33

Chapter 8: Hereditary Neuropathy 38

Chapter 9: Neuropathy Associated with HIV/AIDS................. 43

Chapter 10: Neuropathy Related to Lyme Disease 48

Chapter 11: Alcoholic Neuropathy 53

Chapter 12: Living with Neuropathy: Coping Strategies and Support 58

Chapter 13: Future Directions in Neuropathy Research and Treatment 63

Chapter 14: Conclusion.. 69

Neuropathy Unveiled: Understanding and Managing Diabetic Nerve Damage

By Roberto Miguel Rodriguez

Chapter 1: Introduction to Neuropathy

Understanding Neuropathy

Neuropathy is a term that encompasses a wide range of nerve disorders, each with its own unique symptoms and causes. In this subchapter, we will delve into the various types of neuropathies, shedding light on their distinct characteristics and how they affect individuals. Whether you are living with diabetic neuropathy, peripheral neuropathy, autonomic neuropathy, chemotherapy-induced neuropathy, small fiber neuropathy, idiopathic neuropathy, hereditary neuropathy, neuropathy associated with HIV/AIDS, neuropathy related to Lyme disease, or alcoholic neuropathy, this section will provide valuable insights into your condition.

Diabetic neuropathy is one of the most common forms of neuropathy and is caused by prolonged high blood sugar levels in individuals with diabetes. It primarily affects the feet and legs, leading to numbness, tingling, and pain. Peripheral neuropathy, on the other hand, involves damage to the peripheral nerves that connect the brain and spinal cord to the rest of the body. This condition can cause weakness, numbness, and a loss of coordination.

Autonomic neuropathy affects the nerves that control involuntary bodily functions such as heart rate, digestion, and bladder control. This can result in symptoms like dizziness, digestive issues, and sexual dysfunction. Chemotherapy-induced neuropathy is a side effect of certain cancer treatments that damage the nerves, causing tingling, numbness, and pain in the extremities.

Small fiber neuropathy specifically affects the small nerve fibers responsible for transmitting pain and temperature sensations. This condition often presents a burning sensation and heightened sensitivity to touch. Idiopathic neuropathy refers to cases where the exact cause is unknown and can manifest with a wide range of symptoms.

Hereditary neuropathy is a genetic condition that affects the peripheral nerves, leading to various symptoms depending on the specific gene mutation involved. Neuropathy associated with HIV/AIDS can occur as a result of the virus itself or as a side effect of certain antiretroviral medications. Lyme disease, a tick-borne illness, can also cause neuropathy, resulting in pain, weakness, and numbness. Lastly, alcoholic neuropathy is caused by excessive alcohol consumption over an extended period, leading to nerve damage and symptoms such as muscle weakness and pain.

By understanding the different types of neuropathies, individuals can gain a better grasp of their condition and work towards effective management strategies. It is crucial to consult with healthcare professionals for accurate diagnosis and personalized treatment plans. With the right knowledge and support, individuals can take control of their neuropathy and improve their quality of life.

Causes and Risk Factors of Neuropathy

Neuropathy, a condition characterized by nerve damage, can affect various parts of the body and lead to a wide range of symptoms. Understanding the causes and risk factors of neuropathy is crucial for both prevention and management. In this subchapter, we will delve into the key factors that contribute to different types of neuropathy.

One of the most common types of neuropathy is diabetic neuropathy, which affects individuals with diabetes. Prolonged high blood sugar levels can damage the nerves, leading to symptoms such as numbness, tingling, and pain in the affected areas. It is essential for individuals with diabetes to maintain optimal blood sugar control to reduce the risk of developing neuropathy.

Peripheral neuropathy is another prevalent form of nerve damage that can result from various factors. One of the leading causes is chronic diseases such as diabetes, autoimmune disorders, and kidney disease. Additionally, exposure to toxins, including certain medications, industrial chemicals, and heavy metals, can also contribute to peripheral neuropathy. It is crucial to minimize exposure to such toxins and to consider alternative treatments when possible.

Autonomic neuropathy affects the nerves controlling involuntary bodily functions, such as heart rate, digestion, and blood pressure regulation. Individuals with diabetes are particularly susceptible to this type of neuropathy, as prolonged high blood sugar levels can damage the autonomic nerves. Proper diabetes management, including blood sugar control and regular check-ups, is vital to reduce the risk of autonomic neuropathy.

Chemotherapy-induced neuropathy is a common side effect of cancer treatment. The powerful drugs used in chemotherapy can damage the nerves, leading to symptoms such as pain, numbness, and weakness. While chemotherapy is often necessary to fight cancer, healthcare providers should closely monitor patients and adjust treatment plans to minimize the risk of neuropathy.

Other types of neuropathy, including small fiber neuropathy, idiopathic neuropathy, hereditary neuropathy, neuropathy associated with HIV/AIDS, neuropathy related to Lyme disease, and alcoholic neuropathy, have their own unique causes and risk factors. In-depth knowledge of these factors is essential for accurate diagnosis and effective management.

Overall, understanding the causes and risk factors of neuropathy is crucial for both healthcare providers and individuals. By identifying these factors, we can take proactive steps to prevent or manage neuropathy effectively. From maintaining optimal blood sugar control to minimizing exposure to toxins, each action can make a significant difference in preserving nerve health and improving quality of life.

Impact of Neuropathy on Daily Life

Neuropathy, a condition characterized by nerve damage, can have a profound impact on daily life for individuals suffering from various forms of neuropathy, including diabetic neuropathy, peripheral neuropathy, autonomic neuropathy, chemotherapy-induced neuropathy, small fiber neuropathy, idiopathic neuropathy, hereditary neuropathy, neuropathy associated with HIV/AIDS, neuropathy related to Lyme disease, and alcoholic neuropathy. Understanding the implications of neuropathy on daily life is crucial for both patients and their loved ones.

One of the most significant effects of neuropathy is the disruption it causes to the nervous system, leading to various symptoms that can significantly impair daily activities. Numbness, tingling, and pain in the affected areas, such as the hands and feet, can make simple tasks like walking, grasping objects, and even buttoning a shirt extremely challenging. The constant pain can also disrupt sleep patterns, leading to fatigue and irritability during the day.

Mobility is often severely impacted by neuropathy. Balance issues and muscle weakness can make it difficult for individuals to walk or stand for extended periods. This limitation can greatly affect independence and the ability to perform routine tasks such as grocery shopping, cooking, and cleaning. Additionally, the fear of falling and injuring oneself can lead to social isolation and a decrease in overall quality of life.

Neuropathy can also affect the autonomic nervous system, leading to problems with digestion, bladder control, and blood pressure regulation. Individuals may experience gastrointestinal issues, urinary incontinence, and dizziness, further complicating daily life. These symptoms can be embarrassing and may require adjustments to diet, medication, and lifestyle.

Furthermore, the emotional and psychological toll of living with neuropathy should not be overlooked. Chronic pain and the limitations it imposes can lead to anxiety, depression, and frustration. The constant battle to manage symptoms and maintain a semblance of normalcy can be mentally exhausting, affecting not only the individual but also their relationships with family and friends.

In conclusion, neuropathy has a profound impact on daily life for individuals across various forms, including diabetic neuropathy, peripheral neuropathy, autonomic neuropathy, chemotherapy-induced neuropathy, small fiber neuropathy, idiopathic neuropathy, hereditary neuropathy, neuropathy associated with HIV/AIDS, neuropathy related to Lyme disease, and alcoholic neuropathy. The physical, emotional, and social limitations caused by neuropathy can disrupt routine activities, decrease independence, and negatively affect overall well-being. It is crucial for patients, their loved ones, and the public to understand the challenges faced by those living with neuropathy, in order to provide the necessary support, empathy, and resources to improve their quality of life.

Chapter 2: Diabetic Neuropathy

Overview of Diabetic Neuropathy

Diabetic neuropathy is a common and serious complication that affects individuals with diabetes. It is a type of peripheral neuropathy, which refers to nerve damage that occurs outside of the brain and spinal cord. Diabetic neuropathy can manifest in various forms, including autonomic neuropathy, small fiber neuropathy, and other specific types such as chemotherapy-induced neuropathy, idiopathic neuropathy, hereditary neuropathy, neuropathy associated with HIV/AIDS, neuropathy related to Lyme disease, and alcoholic neuropathy.

Peripheral neuropathy, including diabetic neuropathy, occurs when the nerves responsible for transmitting signals between the central nervous system and the rest of the body become damaged. In the case of diabetic neuropathy, prolonged high blood sugar levels contribute to this nerve damage. Over time, this damage can lead to a range of symptoms that can affect different parts of the body.

Autonomic neuropathy is a specific type of diabetic neuropathy that affects the autonomic nervous system. This system controls involuntary functions such as heart rate, digestion, and blood pressure. Symptoms of autonomic neuropathy can include dizziness, urinary problems, gastrointestinal issues, and sexual dysfunction.

Small fiber neuropathy is another form of diabetic neuropathy that affects the small nerve fibers responsible for detecting pain and temperature changes. Common symptoms include numbness, tingling, and burning sensations in the hands and feet.

Chemotherapy-induced neuropathy is a potential side effect of certain cancer treatments, which can cause nerve damage and lead to symptoms such as numbness, tingling, and weakness in the extremities.

Idiopathic neuropathy refers to cases where the cause of nerve damage is unknown. This form of neuropathy can present with a wide array of symptoms and can be challenging to diagnose and manage.

Hereditary neuropathy is a genetic condition that causes nerve damage and can be passed down through generations. It often affects the peripheral nerves and can lead to symptoms such as muscle weakness, numbness, and pain.

In addition to the specific types mentioned above, neuropathy can also be associated with conditions such as HIV/AIDS and Lyme disease. These infections can damage the nerves and cause symptoms similar to other forms of neuropathy.

Alcoholic neuropathy is a result of excessive alcohol consumption, which can lead to nerve damage. Symptoms may include pain, tingling, and muscle weakness.

Understanding the different types of neuropathy is crucial for both patients and healthcare professionals. By recognizing the specific symptoms and causes, individuals can seek appropriate treatment and management strategies to alleviate pain and prevent further nerve damage.

Symptoms and Progression of Diabetic Neuropathy

Diabetic neuropathy is a common complication of diabetes that affects the nerves throughout the body. It is essential for individuals with diabetes and those who are at risk to understand the symptoms and progression of this condition to effectively manage and minimize its impact on their daily lives.

One of the most common types of diabetic neuropathy is peripheral neuropathy, which primarily affects the nerves in the feet and legs. Symptoms may include tingling, numbness, or pain in the affected areas.

As the condition progresses, individuals may experience a loss of sensation, making it difficult to detect injuries or infections in their lower extremities. This increases the risk of developing foot ulcers, infections, and even amputations if left untreated.

Another type of diabetic neuropathy is autonomic neuropathy, which affects the nerves that control involuntary bodily functions such as digestion, heart rate, and blood pressure. Symptoms may include gastrointestinal problems like nausea, vomiting, and diarrhea, as well as sexual dysfunction, bladder dysfunction, and irregular heart rate. It is important to monitor these symptoms and seek medical attention as they can significantly impact one's quality of life.

Chemotherapy-induced neuropathy is a specific type of neuropathy that can occur as a side effect of certain cancer treatments. Symptoms may include numbness, tingling, or pain in the hands and feet, and it can have a profound impact on an individual's ability to perform daily activities.

Other types of neuropathy, such as small fiber neuropathy, idiopathic neuropathy, hereditary neuropathy, and neuropathy associated with HIV/AIDS or Lyme disease, may have different symptom profiles and progressions. However, the overarching theme is that these conditions can cause significant discomfort and impair daily functioning if not properly managed.

In the book "Neuropathy Unveiled: Understanding and Managing Diabetic Nerve Damage," we delve into each of these specific neuropathies, exploring their symptoms, progression, and available treatment options. By providing valuable information to the public, we aim to empower individuals with knowledge about their condition and encourage them to take an active role in their healthcare.

It is important to remember that early detection and intervention are key in managing neuropathy. Regular check-ups with healthcare professionals and maintaining good blood sugar control can help prevent or delay the onset of neuropathic symptoms. Additionally, adopting a healthy lifestyle, including regular exercise, a balanced diet, and avoiding excessive alcohol consumption, can also contribute to minimizing the progression and impact of neuropathy.

By understanding the symptoms and progression of diabetic neuropathy, individuals can take proactive steps to manage their condition effectively and improve their overall quality of life. "Neuropathy Unveiled" offers a comprehensive guide to help individuals navigate the complexities of diabetic neuropathy and find the best strategies to manage their specific condition, regardless of its underlying cause.

Treatment and Management Options for Diabetic Neuropathy

Diabetic neuropathy is a common complication of diabetes that affects the nerves, leading to a range of symptoms and complications. Fortunately, there are several treatment and management options available to help individuals with diabetic neuropathy lead a better quality of life.

One of the most important aspects of managing diabetic neuropathy is to effectively control blood sugar levels. Maintaining optimal blood glucose levels can slow down the progression of nerve damage and reduce symptoms. This can be achieved through a combination of medication, diet, exercise, and regular monitoring.

Medications can also play a crucial role in managing diabetic neuropathy. Several classes of drugs are commonly prescribed, including antidepressants, anticonvulsants, and opioids. These medications can help relieve pain, improve sleep, and manage other symptoms associated with neuropathy. However, it is important to work closely with a healthcare provider to determine the most appropriate medication and dosage for individual needs.

In addition to medications, various other treatment options can provide relief for diabetic neuropathy. Physical therapy and regular exercise can help improve muscle strength and coordination, reduce pain, and enhance overall mobility. Transcutaneous electrical nerve stimulation (TENS) is another technique that involves using low-level electrical currents to stimulate the nerves and alleviate pain.

Alternative treatments such as acupuncture and massage therapy have also shown promising results in managing diabetic neuropathy. These techniques can help improve blood circulation, reduce pain, and promote relaxation and overall well-being.

Furthermore, lifestyle modifications can significantly impact the management of diabetic neuropathy. Quitting smoking, maintaining a healthy weight, and adopting a balanced diet rich in fruits, vegetables, and whole grains can all contribute to better nerve health and overall diabetes management.

Support groups and counseling can be immensely beneficial for individuals living with diabetic neuropathy. Connecting with others who are facing similar challenges can provide a sense of community and emotional support. It is important to educate oneself about the condition and its management options, empowering individuals to actively participate in their treatment plan and make informed decisions.

While there is currently no cure for diabetic neuropathy, with proper management and treatment, individuals can effectively control symptoms, prevent further nerve damage, and improve their overall quality of life. It is crucial to work closely with healthcare providers to develop a personalized treatment plan that addresses the specific needs and goals of each individual.

This subchapter aims to provide a comprehensive overview of the various treatment and management options available for diabetic neuropathy.

By exploring these options, individuals can gain a better understanding of how to effectively manage their condition and find relief from the symptoms associated with diabetic neuropathy.

Chapter 3: Peripheral Neuropathy

Definition and Types of Peripheral Neuropathy

Peripheral neuropathy is a condition that affects the peripheral nerves, which are the nerves outside the brain and spinal cord. These nerves are responsible for transmitting signals between the body and the central nervous system. When these nerves become damaged or dysfunctional, it can lead to a wide range of symptoms and complications. In this subchapter, we will delve into the definition and various types of peripheral neuropathy, shedding light on the diverse range of conditions that fall under its umbrella.

Diabetic neuropathy is one of the most common types of peripheral neuropathy and occurs in individuals with diabetes. It affects the nerves in the legs and feet, causing symptoms such as numbness, tingling, and pain. Autonomic neuropathy, another type of peripheral neuropathy, affects the nerves that control involuntary bodily functions like digestion, heart rate, and blood pressure. It can lead to complications such as gastrointestinal issues, urinary problems, and cardiovascular abnormalities.

Chemotherapy-induced neuropathy is a consequence of certain cancer treatments, causing damage to the peripheral nerves. This type of neuropathy often results in symptoms such as numbness, tingling, and weakness in the hands and feet. Small fiber neuropathy is characterized by damage to the small nerve fibers, leading to symptoms like burning pain, sensitivity to touch, and changes in temperature perception.

Idiopathic neuropathy refers to cases where the cause of nerve damage is unknown. It can be a frustrating diagnosis, as the underlying cause remains elusive. Hereditary neuropathy is a genetic condition that affects the peripheral nerves, often leading to muscle weakness, loss of sensation, and difficulty with coordination.

Neuropathy associated with HIV/AIDS is a complication of the viral infection, which can damage the peripheral nerves and result in symptoms such as pain, numbness, and muscle weakness. Neuropathy related to Lyme disease occurs due to an infection caused by tick bites and can lead to nerve damage, resulting in symptoms like shooting pain, muscle weakness, and difficulty with balance.

Lastly, alcoholic neuropathy is caused by excessive alcohol consumption and can lead to nerve damage and symptoms such as numbness, tingling, and muscle weakness.

Understanding the various types of peripheral neuropathy is crucial for both patients and the general public. By recognizing the specific characteristics and symptoms of each type, individuals can seek appropriate medical care and management strategies. In the following chapters, we will explore the causes, risk factors, and treatment options for each type of neuropathy, providing valuable knowledge and insights to help individuals effectively manage and cope with these conditions.

Common Causes of Peripheral Neuropathy

Peripheral neuropathy refers to a condition that affects the peripheral nerves, causing pain, numbness, and weakness in various parts of the body. While there are several types of peripheral neuropathy, each with its own unique characteristics, there are some common causes that can lead to the development of this condition. Understanding these causes is crucial for individuals suffering from peripheral neuropathy, as it helps them identify potential risk factors and take necessary precautions.

One of the most prevalent causes of peripheral neuropathy is diabetes, particularly diabetic neuropathy. Diabetes disrupts the body's ability to regulate blood sugar levels, leading to nerve damage over time. This form of neuropathy usually affects the feet and legs, causing symptoms like tingling, burning pain, and loss of sensation.

Chemotherapy-induced neuropathy is another common cause. While chemotherapy is often a life-saving treatment for cancer patients, it can also damage the nerves, resulting in peripheral neuropathy. Patients undergoing chemotherapy may experience symptoms such as numbness, tingling, and muscle weakness in their hands and feet.

Certain infections, such as HIV/AIDS and Lyme disease, can also lead to peripheral neuropathy. The viruses or bacteria associated with these infections can directly damage the peripheral nerves, causing pain, numbness, and muscle weakness.

Alcohol abuse can also contribute to the development of alcoholic neuropathy. Excessive alcohol consumption can lead to vitamin deficiencies, particularly B vitamins, which are essential for healthy nerve function. This deficiency can result in peripheral neuropathy, mainly affecting the extremities.

In some cases, peripheral neuropathy may have no identifiable cause, known as idiopathic neuropathy. This form of neuropathy can be frustrating for patients, as the exact reason for the nerve damage remains unknown. However, with proper management and treatment, the symptoms of idiopathic neuropathy can often be alleviated.

Hereditary neuropathy is another cause of peripheral neuropathy. Certain genetic mutations can affect the structure and function of peripheral nerves, leading to symptoms such as muscle weakness, loss of coordination, and numbness.

Small fiber neuropathy is a specific type of peripheral neuropathy that affects the small nerve fibers responsible for transmitting pain and temperature sensations. It can result from a variety of causes, including diabetes, autoimmune disorders, and certain medications.

Understanding the common causes of peripheral neuropathy is essential for both patients and the general public. By recognizing these causes, individuals can take proactive steps towards prevention, early detection, and effective management of this condition. Whether due to diabetes, chemotherapy, infections, alcohol abuse, or hereditary factors, peripheral neuropathy can have a significant impact on one's quality of life. Therefore, it is crucial to raise awareness and provide support for those affected by this condition.

Diagnosis and Treatment of Peripheral Neuropathy

Peripheral neuropathy, a common condition affecting millions of people worldwide, refers to damage or dysfunction of the peripheral nerves. It is often associated with various underlying causes, including diabetes, chemotherapy, alcoholism, infections, and hereditary factors. Understanding the diagnosis and treatment options for peripheral neuropathy is crucial for individuals who are affected by this condition.

Diagnosing peripheral neuropathy involves a comprehensive evaluation of symptoms, medical history, and physical examination. Patients may experience a range of symptoms, including numbness, tingling, burning sensations, muscle weakness, and loss of coordination. The healthcare provider may also conduct additional tests like nerve conduction studies, electromyography, and blood tests to determine the underlying cause and severity of the neuropathy.

For individuals with diabetic neuropathy, maintaining optimal blood sugar control is crucial to prevent further nerve damage and alleviate symptoms. A combination of lifestyle modifications, such as a healthy diet, regular exercise, and weight management, along with medication management, can help individuals manage their diabetes and reduce the impact on peripheral nerves.

Treatment options for peripheral neuropathy vary depending on the specific cause and severity of the condition. Medications like pain relievers, anti-seizure drugs, and antidepressants are often prescribed to manage pain and other symptoms associated with neuropathy. Physical therapy, occupational therapy, and the use of assistive devices can help improve mobility, balance, and overall quality of life.

In cases of chemotherapy-induced neuropathy, adjustments to the treatment plan may be necessary to minimize nerve damage. Alternative medications and dose modifications can be explored in collaboration with the healthcare team to balance the benefits of chemotherapy with the prevention or management of neuropathy.

Furthermore, individuals with neuropathy associated with HIV/AIDS or Lyme disease require a comprehensive approach that addresses the underlying infection alongside symptomatic management. Antiviral or antibiotic medications may be prescribed, along with supportive care to alleviate neuropathic symptoms.

It is important to note that self-care plays a significant role in managing peripheral neuropathy. Lifestyle modifications, such as quitting smoking, limiting alcohol consumption, protecting the feet from injuries, and practicing good foot hygiene, can help prevent or slow down further nerve damage.

In conclusion, the diagnosis and treatment of peripheral neuropathy require a multi-faceted approach tailored to the underlying cause and individual needs. By working closely with healthcare professionals and adopting self-care strategies, individuals can effectively manage their neuropathy and improve their overall quality of life.

Chapter 4: Autonomic Neuropathy

Understanding Autonomic Neuropathy

Autonomic neuropathy is a type of peripheral neuropathy that affects the autonomic nervous system, which controls the involuntary functions of the body. This condition is often associated with diabetes but can also occur as a result of other factors, such as chemotherapy, alcoholism, or certain genetic conditions.

The autonomic nervous system plays a crucial role in maintaining the body's internal balance, regulating functions such as heart rate, blood pressure, digestion, and temperature control. When the nerves that control these functions are damaged, it can lead to a wide range of symptoms and complications.

In diabetic neuropathy, high blood sugar levels over a prolonged period can damage the nerves throughout the body, including those in the autonomic nervous system. This can result in symptoms such as dizziness upon standing, rapid heart rate, difficulty swallowing, bladder problems, and gastrointestinal issues like bloating, constipation, or diarrhea.

Chemotherapy-induced neuropathy is another common cause of autonomic neuropathy. Certain chemotherapy drugs can damage the nerves, leading to symptoms such as abnormal sweating, changes in blood pressure, and sexual dysfunction.

Small fiber neuropathy is a form of autonomic neuropathy that primarily affects the small nerve fibers responsible for pain and temperature sensation. This can cause symptoms like burning or tingling pain, intolerance to heat or cold, and increased sensitivity to touch.

It is important to note that autonomic neuropathy can also occur as a result of other conditions, such as HIV/AIDS or Lyme disease. In these cases, the underlying infection or immune system dysfunction can damage the nerves, leading to autonomic dysfunction.

Diagnosing autonomic neuropathy involves a thorough medical history, physical examination, and various tests, including nerve conduction studies and autonomic function tests. Treatment focuses on managing symptoms and addressing the underlying cause, if possible. This may involve medications to control blood pressure, regulate heart rate, or manage gastrointestinal symptoms.

In conclusion, autonomic neuropathy is a complex condition that can significantly impact the quality of life for those affected. Understanding the underlying causes and symptoms of autonomic neuropathy is crucial for both patients and healthcare providers to effectively manage this condition. By raising awareness and providing information about autonomic neuropathy, we hope to empower individuals to seek appropriate medical care and improve their overall well-being.

Effects of Autonomic Neuropathy on the Body

Autonomic neuropathy is a condition that affects the autonomic nervous system, which controls many vital functions in the body. It is commonly seen in individuals with diabetes, but can also be caused by other factors such as chemotherapy, alcoholism, HIV/AIDS, Lyme disease, and hereditary or idiopathic factors. Understanding the effects of autonomic neuropathy on the body is crucial for individuals suffering from this condition as well as their loved ones.

One of the most significant impacts of autonomic neuropathy is on the cardiovascular system. The autonomic nervous system controls heart rate, blood pressure, and the constriction and dilation of blood vessels. When this system is compromised, it can result in abnormalities such as orthostatic hypotension, where blood pressure drops upon standing, and tachycardia, an abnormally fast heart rate. These cardiovascular effects can lead to dizziness, fainting, and an increased risk of heart disease.

The gastrointestinal system is also heavily influenced by the autonomic nervous system. Autonomic neuropathy can cause a range of gastrointestinal symptoms, including gastroparesis, a condition where the stomach takes longer to empty its contents. This can lead to symptoms like nausea, vomiting, bloating, and constipation. Additionally, the condition can affect the functioning of the intestines, leading to diarrhea or fecal incontinence.

Autonomic neuropathy can also impact the body's ability to regulate body temperature. The autonomic nervous system helps to control the dilation and constriction of blood vessels in the skin, which aids in heat regulation. When this system is damaged, individuals may experience abnormal sweating patterns, such as excessive sweating or the inability to sweat at all. This can lead to difficulties in tolerating extreme temperatures and an increased risk of heat stroke or hypothermia.

Furthermore, autonomic neuropathy can affect sexual function and bladder control. Both men and women may experience erectile dysfunction or decreased libido as a result of autonomic neuropathy. Additionally, the condition can lead to urinary incontinence or difficulties emptying the bladder completely.

In conclusion, autonomic neuropathy has far-reaching effects on the body, affecting various systems and functions. It is crucial for individuals with autonomic neuropathy and their loved ones to be aware of these effects to better understand and manage the condition. By working closely with healthcare professionals, implementing lifestyle changes, and adhering to treatment plans, individuals can minimize the impact of autonomic neuropathy on their daily lives and overall well-being.

Managing Autonomic Neuropathy Symptoms

Autonomic neuropathy refers to the damage or dysfunction of the autonomic nerves, which control various involuntary bodily functions. This condition can be a result of various underlying causes, including diabetes, chemotherapy, infections, or even genetic factors. The symptoms of autonomic neuropathy can be diverse and affect different parts of the body, making it crucial to understand how to manage them effectively.

One of the most common symptoms of autonomic neuropathy is orthostatic hypotension, which causes a drop in blood pressure upon standing up. To alleviate this symptom, it is recommended to rise slowly from a sitting or lying position, ensuring that you give your body enough time to adjust. Wearing compression stockings can also help improve blood flow and prevent sudden drops in blood pressure.

Gastrointestinal symptoms such as bloating, diarrhea, or constipation can also occur due to autonomic neuropathy. Modifying your diet by incorporating fiber-rich foods, drinking plenty of water, and eating smaller, more frequent meals can help regulate digestion. Additionally, it is advisable to avoid foods that may trigger gastrointestinal discomfort, such as spicy or fatty foods.

Another common symptom is urinary dysfunction, which includes issues such as urinary incontinence or urinary retention. Managing this symptom involves establishing a regular schedule for bathroom visits and practicing pelvic floor exercises to strengthen the muscles responsible for bladder control. In some cases, medication may be necessary to regulate bladder function.

Sexual dysfunction is another aspect of autonomic neuropathy that can significantly impact the quality of life. Open communication with your partner and healthcare provider is crucial to explore available treatment options and find strategies to maintain intimacy and sexual satisfaction.

Medications, devices, or counseling may be recommended to address specific sexual issues.

Moreover, managing autonomic neuropathy symptoms involves maintaining a healthy lifestyle. Regular exercise can improve blood circulation and alleviate symptoms such as numbness or tingling in the extremities. Maintaining a well-balanced diet, monitoring blood sugar levels for those with diabetes, and avoiding smoking and excessive alcohol consumption are also essential steps in managing this condition.

Seeking support from healthcare professionals, joining support groups, or connecting with others who have similar conditions can provide valuable resources and emotional support. Educating yourself about autonomic neuropathy and staying informed about the latest treatment options can empower you to actively participate in your own care.

Remember, managing autonomic neuropathy symptoms is a personalized journey, and what works for one person may not work for another. Collaborating with your healthcare team and adopting a proactive approach to self-care are key to effectively managing the symptoms and improving your overall quality of life.

Chapter 5: Chemotherapy-induced Neuropathy

Overview of Chemotherapy-induced Neuropathy

Chemotherapy is a common treatment for various types of cancer, but it can have unintended side effects, one of which is chemotherapy-induced neuropathy (CIN). This subchapter aims to provide an overview of CIN, explaining what it is and how it can affect individuals undergoing cancer treatment.

Chemotherapy-induced neuropathy refers to nerve damage caused by chemotherapy drugs. These drugs, which are designed to kill cancer cells, can also damage healthy nerves, leading to a range of symptoms. The severity of CIN can vary from person to person, with some experiencing mild symptoms while others may face significant challenges.

The symptoms of CIN can manifest in different ways, depending on the nerves affected. Common symptoms include tingling, numbness, and a burning sensation in the hands and feet. Some individuals may also experience muscle weakness, difficulty with coordination, and changes in reflexes. These symptoms can significantly impact an individual's quality of life, making it difficult to perform everyday tasks and affecting their overall well-being.

It is important for individuals undergoing chemotherapy to be aware of the potential risk of CIN, as early detection and intervention can help manage the symptoms and prevent further progression. Patients should communicate any changes or symptoms they experience to their healthcare team promptly. Additionally, healthcare providers can monitor nerve function through various tests, such as nerve conduction studies or electromyography.

Managing CIN involves a multidisciplinary approach, with the goal of alleviating symptoms and improving quality of life. Treatment options may include medications to control pain and discomfort, physical therapy to improve muscle strength and coordination, and occupational therapy to help individuals adapt to limitations caused by CIN.

Furthermore, individuals can take proactive steps to minimize the risk of developing CIN by adopting a healthy lifestyle. This includes maintaining a balanced diet, engaging in regular exercise, and avoiding alcohol and tobacco use. Additionally, protecting the hands and feet from extreme temperatures and injuries can also reduce the risk of nerve damage.

In conclusion, chemotherapy-induced neuropathy is a potential side effect of cancer treatment that can have a significant impact on an individual's well-being. Being aware of the symptoms, seeking prompt medical attention, and adopting a healthy lifestyle can help manage CIN and improve the overall quality of life for those undergoing chemotherapy.

Risk Factors and Prevention of Chemotherapy-induced Neuropathy

Chemotherapy-induced neuropathy is a potential side effect of certain cancer treatments that can cause damage to the peripheral nerves, leading to symptoms such as numbness, tingling, weakness, and pain in the hands and feet. While this condition is commonly associated with cancer patients, it is crucial to understand the risk factors and preventive measures applicable to the broader public.

One of the primary risk factors for developing chemotherapy-induced neuropathy is the specific chemotherapy drugs used during treatment. Some drugs are more likely to cause nerve damage than others, and the cumulative dose received also plays a significant role. Other risk factors include age, pre-existing neuropathy or nerve damage, and a history of heavy alcohol consumption.

Prevention is key when it comes to managing chemotherapy-induced neuropathy. The first step is to discuss potential nerve damage risks with your oncologist before starting treatment. They may be able to modify your chemotherapy regimen or recommend alternative drugs that are less likely to cause neuropathy. It is also essential to closely monitor the cumulative dose of chemotherapy drugs received, as exceeding certain thresholds may increase the likelihood of developing neuropathy.

Taking care of your overall health can also help reduce the risk and severity of chemotherapy-induced neuropathy. Maintaining a healthy lifestyle, including regular exercise and a well-balanced diet, can improve nerve health and reduce inflammation. Additionally, managing underlying conditions such as diabetes or high blood pressure can minimize the risk of developing peripheral neuropathy.

During chemotherapy treatment, it is crucial to be vigilant about any changes in sensation or nerve-related symptoms. Promptly reporting these symptoms to your healthcare provider allows for early intervention and potential adjustments to your treatment plan. Certain medications, such as nerve pain medications or antioxidants, may be prescribed to alleviate symptoms and prevent further nerve damage.

In conclusion, understanding the risk factors and preventive measures for chemotherapy-induced neuropathy is crucial for those undergoing cancer treatment. By working closely with your healthcare team and adopting a proactive approach to your health, you can minimize the risk of developing this debilitating condition. Remember, early detection and timely intervention are vital in managing chemotherapy-induced neuropathy effectively.

Coping with Chemotherapy-induced Neuropathy

Chemotherapy-induced neuropathy is a common side effect of cancer treatment that can cause significant discomfort and challenges for patients. This subchapter aims to provide information, tips, and coping strategies for individuals dealing with this specific type of neuropathy.

Chemotherapy drugs are powerful medications used to target and destroy cancer cells. However, these drugs can also damage the nerves in the process, leading to symptoms such as pain, numbness, tingling, weakness, and balance issues. Coping with chemotherapy-induced neuropathy requires a multi-faceted approach that involves both medical interventions and self-care techniques.

First and foremost, it is crucial for patients to communicate openly with their healthcare team about their symptoms. Your medical professionals can help monitor and manage your neuropathy, adjusting your treatment plan if necessary. They may also recommend medications or other interventions to alleviate the discomfort associated with neuropathy.

In addition to medical management, self-care plays a vital role in coping with chemotherapy-induced neuropathy. Maintaining a healthy lifestyle is essential, including regular exercise, a balanced diet, and adequate sleep. Physical activity, such as walking or gentle stretching, can help improve circulation and reduce neuropathic symptoms.

Furthermore, managing stress is crucial for coping with neuropathy. Engaging in relaxation techniques like deep breathing, meditation, or yoga can help reduce stress levels and promote overall well-being. Support groups and counseling may also provide an outlet for emotional support and guidance during this challenging time.

Practicing good foot care is particularly important for individuals with chemotherapy-induced neuropathy. Inspect your feet regularly for any injuries or abnormalities, and keep them clean and moisturized. Wearing comfortable, well-fitting shoes and avoiding high heels can prevent further damage to your feet.

Finally, alternative therapies such as acupuncture, massage, and transcutaneous electrical nerve stimulation (TENS) may offer relief for some individuals. It is essential to discuss these options with your healthcare provider to ensure they are safe and appropriate for your specific situation.

Coping with chemotherapy-induced neuropathy can be a challenging journey, but with the right support and self-care strategies, it is possible to manage the symptoms and enhance your quality of life. Remember, you are not alone in this experience, and reaching out for help from healthcare professionals, support groups, and loved ones can make a significant difference in your coping process.

This subchapter also serves as a reminder that there are various other types of neuropathy beyond chemotherapy-induced neuropathy, such as diabetic neuropathy, peripheral neuropathy, and autonomic neuropathy. While the causes and treatments may differ, the coping strategies and self-care techniques discussed here can also be applicable to those living with other forms of neuropathy. Understanding and managing neuropathy, regardless of its origin, is crucial for anyone dealing with the challenges it presents.

Chapter 6: Small Fiber Neuropathy

Definition and Characteristics of Small Fiber Neuropathy

Small fiber neuropathy, also known as SFN, is a type of peripheral neuropathy that affects the small nerve fibers responsible for transmitting pain and temperature sensations. It is a condition that can occur in various contexts, including diabetes, chemotherapy, or even with no identifiable cause. Understanding the definition and characteristics of small fiber neuropathy is crucial for individuals affected by this condition, as well as those who are interested in learning more about neuropathy in general.

Small fiber neuropathy is often associated with diabetes, a chronic disease that affects the body's ability to regulate blood sugar levels. In diabetic neuropathy, high blood sugar levels over time can damage the nerves, including the small fibers. These small nerves are responsible for transmitting sensations from the skin, such as pain, heat, and cold. When damaged, they can cause a range of symptoms, including tingling, burning pain, numbness, and hypersensitivity to touch.

What makes small fiber neuropathy unique is that it predominantly affects the small nerve fibers, which are thinner and more delicate compared to the larger nerve fibers. This means that symptoms may be more specific and localized, often involving the hands and feet. However, in some cases, the symptoms can spread to other parts of the body.

Small fiber neuropathy can also occur as a result of chemotherapy, where certain medications used to treat cancer can damage the nerve fibers. Additionally, it can be idiopathic, meaning that the cause is unknown, or hereditary, passed down through generations. Other conditions, such as HIV/AIDS or Lyme disease, can also lead to small fiber neuropathy due to the impact they have on the nervous system.

Diagnosing small fiber neuropathy typically involves a thorough medical history review, physical examination, and specialized tests like skin biopsies or nerve conduction studies. Early detection is crucial to prevent complications and manage symptoms effectively.

Treatment for small fiber neuropathy focuses on managing the underlying cause, if known, and providing symptomatic relief. Medications such as pain relievers, antidepressants, and anticonvulsants may be prescribed to help manage pain and improve quality of life. Lifestyle modifications, including regular exercise, a healthy diet, and stress management techniques, can also play a significant role in managing symptoms.

In conclusion, small fiber neuropathy is a type of peripheral neuropathy that primarily affects the small nerve fibers responsible for transmitting pain and temperature sensations. It can occur in various contexts, including diabetes, chemotherapy, or without an identifiable cause. Understanding the definition and characteristics of small fiber neuropathy is essential for individuals affected by this condition, as well as those interested in neuropathy-related topics. Early diagnosis and appropriate treatment can help individuals effectively manage their symptoms and improve their overall quality of life.

Symptoms and Diagnosis of Small Fiber Neuropathy

Small fiber neuropathy (SFN) is a type of peripheral neuropathy that affects the small nerve fibers in the skin and organs. It can be caused by various factors, including diabetes, autoimmune disorders, infections, toxins, and genetic conditions. SFN can result in a range of symptoms and can significantly impact the quality of life for those affected.

The symptoms of SFN can vary from person to person, making it challenging to diagnose. Common symptoms include a burning or tingling sensation, numbness, hypersensitivity to touch, and pain that is often described as sharp or stabbing. These symptoms typically begin in the feet and legs but can also affect the hands and other parts of the body.

In addition to sensory symptoms, SFN can also cause autonomic symptoms. Autonomic neuropathy refers to damage to the nerves that control involuntary bodily functions, such as heart rate, blood pressure, digestion, and sweating. Therefore, individuals with SFN may experience symptoms such as dizziness, rapid heartbeat, digestive problems, abnormal sweating, and bladder dysfunction.

Diagnosing SFN can be challenging, as the symptoms often overlap with other types of neuropathy. A comprehensive medical history, physical examination, and certain tests can help determine if SFN is the underlying cause of the symptoms. These tests may include nerve conduction studies, skin biopsies, autonomic function tests, and blood tests to check for underlying conditions or genetic mutations.

It is essential to seek medical attention if you experience any symptoms of SFN, as early diagnosis and treatment can help manage the condition and prevent further damage. Treatment options for SFN aim to alleviate symptoms and address the underlying cause if possible. This may involve medications to manage pain and improve nerve function, physical therapy to improve balance and strength, and lifestyle modifications to control underlying conditions like diabetes.

It is crucial for individuals with SFN to work closely with their healthcare team to develop an individualized treatment plan and manage their symptoms effectively. Support groups and educational resources can also be valuable in helping individuals cope with the challenges associated with SFN.

In conclusion, small fiber neuropathy is a condition that affects the small nerve fibers in the skin and organs, resulting in a range of sensory and autonomic symptoms. Early diagnosis and treatment are essential for managing the condition and improving quality of life. If you or someone you know experiences symptoms of SFN, it is important to consult with a healthcare professional for proper evaluation and care.

Treatment Approaches for Small Fiber Neuropathy

Small fiber neuropathy (SFN) is a debilitating condition that affects the sensory nerves in the body, resulting in symptoms such as burning pain, tingling, and numbness in the hands and feet. It can be caused by various factors, including diabetes, autoimmune disorders, and certain medications. The treatment approaches for small fiber neuropathy depend on the underlying cause and aim to alleviate symptoms and improve quality of life for patients.

One of the primary treatment approaches for SFN is to address the underlying cause. For instance, in cases where diabetes is the cause, it is crucial to manage blood sugar levels effectively through diet, exercise, and medications. By maintaining stable blood sugar levels, the progression of small fiber neuropathy can be slowed down, and symptoms may improve.

Medications play a vital role in managing the symptoms of small fiber neuropathy. Pain medications such as over-the-counter analgesics and prescription drugs like gabapentin and pregabalin can help alleviate the burning and tingling sensations associated with SFN. However, it is essential to consult a healthcare professional before starting any medication to ensure proper dosage and minimize potential side effects.

In addition to medications, certain lifestyle modifications can also help manage small fiber neuropathy. Regular exercise, such as walking or swimming, can improve blood flow to the nerves and reduce pain. Physical therapy may also be recommended to improve muscle strength and flexibility, which can help compensate for the sensory deficits caused by SFN.

Alternative therapies, such as acupuncture, transcutaneous electrical nerve stimulation (TENS), and biofeedback, have shown promise in relieving pain and improving overall well-being in patients with small fiber neuropathy. These therapies work by stimulating the nerves, promoting relaxation, and reducing stress.

It is important for individuals with small fiber neuropathy to take care of their feet and practice good foot hygiene. Regular foot inspections, proper footwear, and keeping the feet dry and clean can help prevent complications such as infections and foot ulcers.

In conclusion, the treatment approaches for small fiber neuropathy focus on managing the underlying cause, alleviating symptoms, and improving overall quality of life. By effectively managing blood sugar levels, using appropriate medications, adopting a healthy lifestyle, and considering alternative therapies, individuals with small fiber neuropathy can find relief from their symptoms and regain control over their daily lives. Always consult a healthcare professional for personalized advice and guidance in managing small fiber neuropathy.

Chapter 7: Idiopathic Neuropathy

Understanding Idiopathic Neuropathy

Idiopathic neuropathy is a term used to describe a type of nerve damage that occurs without a known cause. It is characterized by the dysfunction or degeneration of the peripheral nerves, which are responsible for transmitting signals between the central nervous system and the rest of the body. This condition can affect individuals of any age, gender, or ethnicity, making it a significant concern for many people.

Idiopathic neuropathy is a diagnosis of exclusion, meaning that it is made when all other possible causes of nerve damage have been ruled out. Medical professionals may conduct a series of tests, including blood work, nerve conduction studies, and imaging, to eliminate other potential causes such as diabetes, autoimmune disorders, or vitamin deficiencies. Once all other possibilities have been excluded, the individual is diagnosed with idiopathic neuropathy.

The exact cause of idiopathic neuropathy remains unknown, which can be frustrating for both patients and healthcare providers. However, it is believed that a combination of genetic, environmental, and lifestyle factors may contribute to the development of this condition. Some studies have suggested that certain individuals may have a genetic predisposition to nerve damage, while others propose that environmental toxins or infections may trigger the onset of symptoms.

The symptoms of idiopathic neuropathy can vary widely from person to person. Common symptoms include tingling or numbness in the extremities, muscle weakness, difficulty walking, and a loss of coordination. In some cases, individuals may also experience pain, burning sensations, or sensitivity to touch. These symptoms can significantly impact a person's quality of life, making it difficult to perform everyday tasks or participate in activities they once enjoyed.

Treatment options for idiopathic neuropathy are limited, as there is no specific cure. However, healthcare providers may recommend a combination of medications, physical therapy, and lifestyle modifications to manage symptoms and slow the progression of nerve damage. Pain management techniques, such as over-the-counter or prescription medications, can help alleviate discomfort. Physical therapy can improve muscle strength and coordination, while lifestyle modifications, such as maintaining a healthy diet and exercising regularly, can promote overall nerve health.

In conclusion, idiopathic neuropathy is a complex condition characterized by nerve damage without a known cause. While the exact mechanisms behind this condition remain unclear, healthcare providers are dedicated to managing symptoms and improving the quality of life for individuals living with this condition. By understanding the nature of idiopathic neuropathy and exploring potential treatment options, individuals can take proactive steps towards managing their symptoms and living a fulfilling life.

Diagnosis and Management of Idiopathic Neuropathy

Idiopathic neuropathy refers to nerve damage that occurs without a known cause. It can be a frustrating condition for both patients and healthcare professionals, as the exact underlying factors are often unclear. In this subchapter, we will delve into the diagnosis and management of idiopathic neuropathy, providing valuable information for individuals suffering from this condition.

Diagnosis is the first step in understanding and managing idiopathic neuropathy. A comprehensive medical history and physical examination are essential to rule out other potential causes of nerve damage. Blood tests may be conducted to check for vitamin deficiencies, thyroid disorders, or autoimmune diseases that could contribute to the neuropathy. Additionally, nerve conduction studies and electromyography may be performed to assess the function of the nerves and muscles. These tests can help determine the extent and location of the nerve damage.

Once diagnosed, the management of idiopathic neuropathy focuses on alleviating symptoms and preventing further damage. A multidisciplinary approach involving healthcare professionals from various specialties is often beneficial. Pain management may involve the use of medications such as antidepressants, anticonvulsants, and opioids. Physical therapy can help improve muscle strength and coordination, while occupational therapy can assist with daily activities affected by neuropathy.

Lifestyle modifications play a crucial role in managing idiopathic neuropathy. Maintaining a healthy diet rich in essential nutrients, especially vitamins B12 and D, can support nerve health. Regular exercise, such as walking or swimming, can improve circulation and reduce neuropathic pain. Quitting smoking and limiting alcohol consumption are also important, as both can exacerbate nerve damage.

In addition to these general management strategies, individuals with idiopathic neuropathy should closely monitor their symptoms and communicate any changes to their healthcare providers. Regular check-ups are essential to track progress and adjust treatment plans accordingly. Support groups and online communities can provide a valuable source of emotional support and information exchange among individuals facing similar challenges.

In conclusion, the diagnosis and management of idiopathic neuropathy require a comprehensive approach that involves medical professionals, lifestyle modifications, and patient education. Although the exact cause may remain unknown, individuals can take proactive steps to alleviate symptoms and improve their quality of life. By understanding the importance of early diagnosis and adopting a multidisciplinary approach, those with idiopathic neuropathy can navigate their condition with confidence and hope for a better future.

Research and Future Directions for Idiopathic Neuropathy

Idiopathic neuropathy refers to a form of peripheral neuropathy where the cause remains unknown. This condition can be frustrating for both patients and healthcare professionals, as the lack of a clear cause makes it challenging to develop targeted treatment approaches. However, ongoing research and future directions in the field of idiopathic neuropathy hold promise for improved understanding and management of this condition.

One area of research focuses on identifying potential underlying mechanisms behind idiopathic neuropathy. Scientists are investigating various factors that could contribute to the development of this condition, including genetic predispositions, autoimmune responses, and inflammatory processes. By unraveling these mechanisms, researchers hope to develop more effective treatments that can target the root cause of idiopathic neuropathy.

Another promising avenue of research involves the use of advanced diagnostic techniques. In recent years, technological advancements have allowed for more precise identification and characterization of nerve damage. These techniques include nerve conduction studies, electromyography, skin biopsy, and autonomic function tests. By employing these tools, healthcare professionals can gain a better understanding of the specific nerve fibers affected in idiopathic neuropathy, which can help in tailoring treatment strategies accordingly.

Furthermore, clinical trials are being conducted to explore novel treatment options for idiopathic neuropathy. These trials assess the safety and effectiveness of various medications, including immunosuppressants, intravenous immunoglobulin therapy, and nerve growth factors. Additionally, alternative therapies such as acupuncture, physical therapy, and transcutaneous electrical nerve stimulation (TENS) are also under investigation. The goal is to find interventions that can alleviate symptoms, improve quality of life, and potentially slow down or halt the progression of idiopathic neuropathy.

It is essential for individuals with idiopathic neuropathy to actively participate in research studies and clinical trials. By doing so, they can contribute to the advancement of knowledge in this field and potentially benefit from emerging treatment options. Additionally, engaging in support groups and patient advocacy organizations can provide valuable insights and create a sense of community among those affected by this condition.

While much progress has been made, the future of idiopathic neuropathy research holds immense potential. With continued efforts, it is hoped that a clearer understanding of the causes and mechanisms behind this condition will emerge, leading to more targeted treatments and improved outcomes for individuals living with idiopathic neuropathy.

Chapter 8: Hereditary Neuropathy

Overview of Hereditary Neuropathy

Hereditary neuropathy refers to a group of genetic disorders that affect the peripheral nerves, resulting in nerve damage and dysfunction. Unlike other forms of neuropathy, hereditary neuropathy is passed down through families and can be present from birth or develop later in life.

One of the most well-known types of hereditary neuropathy is Charcot-Marie-Tooth disease (CMT), which affects both motor and sensory nerves. CMT is characterized by muscle weakness, loss of sensation, and foot deformities. It is estimated that 1 in every 2,500 people is affected by CMT worldwide.

Another type of hereditary neuropathy is hereditary sensory and autonomic neuropathy (HSAN), which primarily affects the sensory and autonomic nerves. HSAN can result in a loss of pain and temperature sensation, as well as problems with sweating, digestion, and blood pressure regulation.

Hereditary neuropathy can be further classified into different subtypes, each with its own unique symptoms and genetic mutations. These subtypes include hereditary motor neuropathy, hereditary sensory neuropathy, and hereditary sensory and motor neuropathy.

Diagnosing hereditary neuropathy can be challenging, as symptoms can vary widely and overlap with other forms of neuropathy. Genetic testing is often used to confirm a diagnosis and identify the specific gene mutation responsible for the condition.

Unfortunately, there is currently no cure for hereditary neuropathy. Treatment focuses on managing symptoms and preventing complications. This may include physical therapy to improve muscle strength and coordination, medications to alleviate pain and neuropathic symptoms, and assistive devices to aid with mobility.

It is important for individuals with hereditary neuropathy to work closely with healthcare professionals, including neurologists and genetic counselors, to develop a personalized treatment plan and address any potential complications.

While hereditary neuropathy is a rare condition, it is essential for the public to be aware of its existence, especially those with a family history of the disease. Early detection and intervention can significantly improve the quality of life for individuals living with hereditary neuropathy.

In conclusion, hereditary neuropathy is a group of genetic disorders that affect the peripheral nerves, leading to nerve damage and dysfunction. With various subtypes and symptoms, hereditary neuropathy requires a multidisciplinary approach to diagnosis and management. Although there is no cure, early detection and appropriate treatment can help individuals with hereditary neuropathy live fulfilling lives.

Common Types of Hereditary Neuropathy

Hereditary neuropathy refers to a group of inherited disorders that affect the peripheral nerves, resulting in various symptoms such as numbness, tingling, weakness, and pain. These conditions are caused by genetic mutations that disrupt the normal functioning of the nerves. Understanding the different types of hereditary neuropathy can help individuals and their families recognize the signs and seek appropriate medical care.

One of the most prevalent types of hereditary neuropathy is Charcot-Marie-Tooth disease (CMT). CMT affects both motor and sensory nerves, leading to muscle weakness and loss of sensation in the extremities. This condition is usually diagnosed in adolescence or early adulthood and can vary in severity. CMT is caused by mutations in genes that are responsible for the production of proteins essential for nerve function.

Another form of hereditary neuropathy is hereditary sensory and autonomic neuropathy (HSAN). HSAN primarily affects the sensory and autonomic nerves, leading to a loss of pain sensation, temperature regulation issues, and problems with the sweat glands. There are several subtypes of HSAN, each caused by different genetic mutations. The severity and specific symptoms can vary widely between individuals.

Friedreich's ataxia is yet another type of hereditary neuropathy. This condition affects both the peripheral nerves and the central nervous system. Individuals with Friedreich's ataxia may experience muscle weakness, difficulty with coordination, and impaired speech. Friedreich's ataxia is caused by a mutation in the frataxin gene, which leads to a deficiency of this important protein.

Other types of hereditary neuropathy include hereditary sensory neuropathy (HSN), hereditary motor neuropathy (HMN), and familial amyloid polyneuropathy (FAP). Each of these conditions has its own specific set of symptoms and genetic causes.

While hereditary neuropathies cannot currently be cured, there are various treatments available to manage the symptoms and slow down the progression of the disease. Physical therapy, pain management techniques, assistive devices, and medications can all be used to improve quality of life for individuals with hereditary neuropathy.

If you suspect that you or a loved one may have hereditary neuropathy, it is crucial to seek medical attention. A thorough evaluation by a neurologist or geneticist can help determine the specific type of hereditary neuropathy and guide appropriate treatment options.

In summary, hereditary neuropathies encompass a range of inherited disorders that affect the peripheral nerves. Recognizing the common types of hereditary neuropathy, such as Charcot-Marie-Tooth disease, hereditary sensory and autonomic neuropathy, and Friedreich's ataxia, can help individuals and their families understand the symptoms and seek appropriate medical care. While there is currently no cure for hereditary neuropathy, various treatments can help manage the symptoms and improve quality of life.

Genetic Testing and Treatment Options for Hereditary Neuropathy

In our quest to better understand and manage neuropathy, it is crucial to explore the genetic aspects of this condition. Genetic testing has emerged as a powerful tool in identifying hereditary neuropathy and tailoring treatment options for individuals affected by this form of the disorder. Hereditary neuropathy is a distinct subset of neuropathy, characterized by its inheritance pattern and the specific genetic mutations involved.

Advancements in genetic testing have revolutionized the field of medicine, enabling healthcare providers to identify specific genetic mutations responsible for hereditary neuropathy. By pinpointing the genetic cause, doctors can provide accurate diagnoses, offer personalized treatment plans, and even predict the likelihood of passing on the condition to future generations.

Identifying the genetic mutations associated with hereditary neuropathy not only aids in diagnosis but also helps guide treatment decisions. Different genetic mutations can lead to variations in symptoms, disease progression, and response to treatment. With genetic testing, healthcare providers can develop targeted therapies that address the underlying cause of the neuropathy, potentially improving outcomes for patients.

Furthermore, genetic testing plays a vital role in genetic counseling. It allows individuals and families at risk of hereditary neuropathy to make informed decisions about family planning and understand the likelihood of passing on the condition to their children. Genetic counseling can provide emotional support, facilitate informed decision-making, and help individuals navigate the complexities of hereditary neuropathy.

While genetic testing offers valuable insights, it is important to note that not all forms of neuropathy are hereditary. Other factors, such as diabetes, chemotherapy, or infections, can also contribute to the development of neuropathy. Therefore, it is crucial to consider a comprehensive approach to diagnosing and managing neuropathy, taking into account both genetic and environmental factors.

In conclusion, genetic testing has revolutionized our understanding and management of hereditary neuropathy. By identifying specific genetic mutations, healthcare providers can offer tailored treatment options, predict disease progression, and provide genetic counseling. However, it is essential to recognize that not all neuropathies are hereditary, and a comprehensive approach is necessary to address the various causes of neuropathy effectively. By combining genetic testing with other diagnostic tools and approaches, we can strive towards better outcomes for individuals affected by all forms of neuropathy.

Chapter 9: Neuropathy Associated with HIV/AIDS

HIV/AIDS-related Neuropathy Explained

HIV/AIDS is a global health concern that affects millions of people worldwide. While most commonly known for its impact on the immune system, HIV/AIDS can also lead to a variety of other complications, including neuropathy. In this subchapter, we will delve into the specific details of HIV/AIDS-related neuropathy and its implications for those living with the virus.

Neuropathy refers to damage or dysfunction of the nerves, resulting in a wide range of symptoms such as numbness, tingling, pain, and weakness. When it comes to HIV/AIDS, neuropathy can develop as a direct result of the virus or as a side effect of antiretroviral medications used to treat it.

HIV/AIDS-related neuropathy typically affects the peripheral nervous system, which includes the nerves outside of the brain and spinal cord. It often presents as a distal symmetric polyneuropathy, meaning it affects both sides of the body symmetrically, starting in the feet and gradually moving upwards. Common symptoms include a loss of sensation, burning or shooting pain, muscle weakness, and difficulty with coordination.

The exact mechanisms behind HIV/AIDS-related neuropathy are not fully understood. However, it is believed that the virus itself may directly damage the nerves, while medications used to manage the infection can also contribute to nerve damage. Additionally, other factors such as inflammation, immune system dysfunction, and nutritional deficiencies may play a role in the development of neuropathy in individuals living with HIV/AIDS.

Managing HIV/AIDS-related neuropathy involves a multi-faceted approach. Firstly, it is crucial to effectively control the underlying HIV infection with antiretroviral therapy. This not only helps to slow down the progression of neuropathy but also improves overall health and quality of life. Additionally, symptomatic relief can be achieved through various medications, including pain relievers, antidepressants, and anticonvulsants.

Non-pharmacological interventions such as physical therapy, occupational therapy, and alternative therapies like acupuncture and nerve stimulation techniques may also be beneficial in managing the symptoms of HIV/AIDS-related neuropathy. It is important to work closely with a healthcare team to develop an individualized treatment plan that addresses the specific needs and concerns of each person.

In conclusion, HIV/AIDS-related neuropathy is a significant complication of the virus that can greatly impact the quality of life for those affected. Understanding the causes, symptoms, and management strategies for this condition is crucial for individuals living with HIV/AIDS, as well as their healthcare providers. By taking a comprehensive approach and addressing the underlying infection while effectively managing symptoms, individuals can strive for a better quality of life despite the challenges presented by HIV/AIDS-related neuropathy.

Symptoms and Progression of Neuropathy in HIV/AIDS

Neuropathy is a common complication of HIV/AIDS, affecting a significant number of individuals living with the disease. Understanding the symptoms and progression of neuropathy in the context of HIV/AIDS is crucial for both patients and healthcare professionals. In this subchapter, we will explore the various aspects of neuropathy associated with HIV/AIDS, including its symptoms, progression, and potential management strategies.

Neuropathy refers to nerve damage or dysfunction that can disrupt the normal functioning of the peripheral nervous system. In the case of HIV/AIDS, neuropathy can occur due to multiple factors, including the direct impact of the virus on nerve cells, the side effects of antiretroviral medications, and the weakened immune system's vulnerability to opportunistic infections.

The symptoms of neuropathy in individuals with HIV/AIDS can vary depending on the specific type of nerve fibers affected. Some common symptoms include tingling, numbness, and a burning sensation in the extremities, such as the hands and feet. Muscle weakness, difficulty with coordination, and balance problems may also occur. Moreover, individuals may experience sharp or shooting pain, which can be debilitating and greatly impact their quality of life.

The progression of neuropathy in HIV/AIDS is often gradual, starting with mild symptoms that may be ignored or attributed to other factors. As the disease progresses, however, the symptoms tend to worsen and can even spread to other parts of the body. In some cases, the autonomic nervous system may be affected, leading to symptoms such as dizziness upon standing, abnormal heart rate, and gastrointestinal issues.

Managing neuropathy in the context of HIV/AIDS requires a comprehensive approach. Firstly, it is crucial to address the underlying HIV infection itself through appropriate antiretroviral therapy. This can help slow down the progression of neuropathy and prevent further damage to the nerves. Additionally, managing pain and discomfort is essential, and medications such as analgesics, antidepressants, and anticonvulsants may be prescribed to alleviate symptoms.

Beyond medication, lifestyle modifications can play a significant role in managing neuropathy. Regular exercise, a healthy diet, and avoiding alcohol and tobacco can help improve overall nerve health. Physical therapy and occupational therapy may also be beneficial in improving mobility and managing daily activities.

In conclusion, neuropathy associated with HIV/AIDS can significantly impact the lives of individuals living with the disease. Recognizing the symptoms and understanding the progression of neuropathy is essential for early detection and effective management. By addressing the underlying HIV infection, managing symptoms, and adopting a holistic approach to care, individuals can improve their quality of life and minimize the impact of neuropathy on their overall well-being.

Managing Neuropathy in HIV/AIDS Patients

Neuropathy is a condition characterized by damage to the nerves, leading to a range of symptoms such as numbness, tingling, and pain. While it is commonly associated with diabetes, there are several other underlying causes, including HIV/AIDS. In this subchapter, we will explore how to effectively manage neuropathy in HIV/AIDS patients.

Neuropathy associated with HIV/AIDS is a complex condition that requires a comprehensive approach to treatment. The first step in managing this type of neuropathy is to address the underlying HIV infection. Antiretroviral therapy (ART) is crucial in controlling the virus and preventing further nerve damage. By effectively managing HIV/AIDS, the progression of neuropathy can be slowed or even halted.

Additionally, pain management plays a vital role in enhancing the quality of life for individuals with HIV/AIDS-related neuropathy. Non-opioid pain medications, such as over-the-counter pain relievers, can help alleviate mild to moderate pain. However, in cases of severe pain, stronger medications may be necessary and should be prescribed by a healthcare professional.

Physical therapy can also be beneficial in managing neuropathy symptoms. Engaging in regular exercise and physical activities can improve blood circulation and reduce pain. It is important to consult with a physical therapist to determine the most appropriate exercises for each individual's unique needs.

Furthermore, adopting a healthy lifestyle is crucial in managing neuropathy associated with HIV/AIDS. This includes maintaining a balanced diet, quitting smoking, moderating alcohol consumption, and managing stress levels. These lifestyle changes can significantly contribute to the overall well-being of individuals with neuropathy.

Support groups and counseling can provide tremendous emotional support for those living with HIV/AIDS-related neuropathy. Connecting with others who are experiencing similar challenges can offer a sense of understanding and camaraderie. Additionally, counseling can help individuals cope with the emotional and psychological impact of living with a chronic condition.

In conclusion, managing neuropathy in HIV/AIDS patients requires a multidimensional approach. By effectively managing the underlying HIV infection, utilizing pain management techniques, engaging in physical therapy, adopting a healthy lifestyle, and seeking emotional support, individuals can experience improved quality of life. It is important to work closely with healthcare professionals to develop a personalized treatment plan that addresses the unique needs of each individual living with neuropathy associated with HIV/AIDS.

Chapter 10: Neuropathy Related to Lyme Disease

Lyme Disease and its Impact on Nerve Health

Lyme disease is a bacterial infection caused by the bite of an infected black-legged tick. While the disease primarily affects the skin, joints, and heart, it can also have a significant impact on nerve health. In this subchapter, we will explore the connection between Lyme disease and neuropathy, shedding light on the potential risks and complications associated with this tick-borne illness.

Neuropathy is a condition characterized by damage to the nerves, leading to a variety of symptoms such as numbness, tingling, and pain. Among the various types of neuropathy, Lyme disease-related neuropathy is a lesser-known but important consideration for those living in or traveling to areas infested with ticks.

When Lyme disease bacteria enter the body through a tick bite, they can trigger an immune response that inadvertently damages the nerves. This immune response, known as neuroborreliosis, often manifests as peripheral neuropathy, affecting the nerves outside of the brain and spinal cord. Symptoms may include weakness, sensory disturbances, and muscle pain.

In some cases, Lyme disease can also lead to autonomic neuropathy, which affects the nerves controlling involuntary bodily functions such as heart rate, blood pressure, and digestion. This can result in symptoms like dizziness, irregular heartbeats, and difficulty swallowing.

It is essential to note that Lyme disease-related neuropathy can be challenging to diagnose, as its symptoms can mimic those of other conditions. Therefore, individuals who have been exposed to ticks or live in high-risk areas should be vigilant and seek medical attention if they experience any unusual neurological symptoms.

Managing Lyme disease-related neuropathy involves a multifaceted approach. Antibiotics are the primary treatment for Lyme disease itself, which can help alleviate the underlying infection and, consequently, reduce the impact on nerve health. Additionally, symptomatic relief can be achieved through medications targeting neuropathic pain, physical therapy, and lifestyle modifications to improve overall nerve health.

Prevention is equally crucial in combating Lyme disease-related neuropathy. This includes employing tick repellents, wearing protective clothing when outdoors, thoroughly checking for and removing ticks after potential exposure, and staying informed about the prevalence of Lyme disease in your area.

By understanding the connection between Lyme disease and neuropathy, individuals can take proactive measures to protect their nerve health. With early detection, appropriate treatment, and preventive strategies, the impact of Lyme disease on nerve health can be minimized, promoting overall well-being for those affected by this tick-borne illness.

Recognizing and Diagnosing Lyme Disease-related Neuropathy

Lyme disease is a tick-borne illness caused by the bacteria Borrelia burgdorferi. While it is commonly associated with joint pain and flu-like symptoms, many people are unaware that it can also lead to neuropathy, a condition characterized by damage to the nerves. Lyme disease-related neuropathy can cause a wide range of symptoms, making it crucial to recognize and diagnose the condition early on for effective management.

One of the first signs of Lyme disease-related neuropathy is often tingling or numbness in the extremities, such as the hands and feet. These sensations may come and go, making it easy to dismiss them as temporary discomfort. However, if left untreated, the neuropathy can progress and lead to more severe symptoms, including sharp or burning pain, muscle weakness, and even difficulty walking.

Diagnosing Lyme disease-related neuropathy can be challenging, as its symptoms can mimic those of other types of neuropathy. However, doctors will typically consider several factors when making a diagnosis. A thorough medical history, including any recent exposure to ticks or outdoor activities in areas where Lyme disease is prevalent, is essential. Additionally, blood tests can be conducted to check for the presence of Lyme disease antibodies.

It is important to note that Lyme disease-related neuropathy may not always be accompanied by the characteristic bullseye rash associated with Lyme disease. In fact, many individuals with Lyme disease-related neuropathy may not even recall being bitten by a tick. Therefore, it is crucial to be aware of the possibility of Lyme disease-related neuropathy, even in the absence of these typical symptoms.

Once diagnosed, managing Lyme disease-related neuropathy involves a multifaceted approach. Antibiotics are the primary treatment for Lyme disease itself, and early treatment greatly improves the chances of preventing complications like neuropathy. Pain management strategies, such as medications and physical therapy, may be recommended to alleviate symptoms.

Prevention is key when it comes to Lyme disease-related neuropathy. Taking precautions to avoid tick bites, such as wearing protective clothing and using insect repellents, is essential, especially when spending time in wooded or grassy areas. Performing regular tick checks and promptly removing any ticks found can also help prevent the transmission of Lyme disease.

In conclusion, recognizing and diagnosing Lyme disease-related neuropathy is vital for effective management and prevention of complications. Understanding the potential symptoms and risk factors associated with this condition allows individuals to seek medical attention promptly. By taking preventive measures and seeking early treatment, individuals can minimize the impact of Lyme disease-related neuropathy on their overall well-being.

Treatment Approaches for Lyme Disease-related Neuropathy

Lyme disease is a tick-borne illness caused by the bacteria Borrelia burgdorferi. While most commonly associated with joint pain and flu-like symptoms, Lyme disease can also lead to neuropathy, a condition characterized by damage to the nerves. When Lyme disease affects the peripheral nervous system, it can cause a range of symptoms, including numbness, tingling, muscle weakness, and shooting pains.

Treating Lyme disease-related neuropathy requires a comprehensive approach that targets both the underlying infection and the symptoms of nerve damage. Here are some treatment approaches that have shown promise in managing this condition:

1. Antibiotics: Since Lyme disease is caused by a bacterial infection, antibiotics are the primary treatment. Oral or intravenous antibiotics may be prescribed depending on the severity of the infection. It is crucial to complete the full course of antibiotics as prescribed by your healthcare provider to effectively eliminate the bacteria.

2. Pain management: Lyme disease-related neuropathy can cause significant discomfort. Pain medications, such as nonsteroidal anti-inflammatory drugs (NSAIDs) or opioids, may be prescribed to alleviate pain. Additionally, topical treatments, such as lidocaine patches, can provide localized relief.

3. Physical therapy: Physical therapy can help improve muscle strength, flexibility, and balance, which can be compromised by neuropathy. A

physical therapist can design an exercise program tailored to your specific needs and abilities.

4. Nerve stimulation: Certain types of neuropathy may benefit from nerve stimulation techniques. Transcutaneous electrical nerve stimulation (TENS) uses low-voltage electrical currents to provide pain relief by blocking nerve signals. Other forms of nerve stimulation, such as spinal cord stimulation, may be considered for severe or chronic cases.

5. Complementary therapies: Some individuals find relief from complementary therapies, such as acupuncture, massage, or chiropractic care. These therapies can help reduce pain and promote relaxation, though their effectiveness may vary from person to person.

6. Supportive care: Managing Lyme disease-related neuropathy involves not only treating the physical symptoms but also addressing the emotional and psychological impact. Support groups, counseling, and stress management techniques can play a crucial role in helping individuals cope with the challenges posed by chronic neuropathy.

It is important to consult with a healthcare professional experienced in treating Lyme disease-related neuropathy to develop a personalized treatment plan. They can assess your specific condition, consider any other underlying medical issues, and guide you through the various treatment options available. With the right approach, it is possible to manage Lyme disease-related neuropathy and improve the quality of life for those affected.

Chapter 11: Alcoholic Neuropathy

Alcohol Abuse and its Effects on Nerve Function

Introduction:

Alcohol abuse is a prevalent issue in society that affects millions of individuals worldwide. It not only poses a threat to physical and mental health but can also have severe consequences on nerve function. In this subchapter, we will explore the detrimental effects of alcohol abuse on various types of neuropathy, including diabetic neuropathy, peripheral neuropathy, autonomic neuropathy, chemotherapy-induced neuropathy, small fiber neuropathy, idiopathic neuropathy, hereditary neuropathy, neuropathy associated with HIV/AIDS, neuropathy related to Lyme disease, and alcoholic neuropathy.

Alcoholic Neuropathy:

Alcoholic neuropathy is a specific type of neuropathy caused by excessive and prolonged alcohol consumption. Chronic alcohol abuse can lead to damage to the peripheral nerves, resulting in symptoms such as numbness, tingling, and pain in the extremities. This condition often starts with sensory symptoms in the toes and feet, gradually progressing to the hands and fingers.

Impact on Diabetic Neuropathy:

For individuals already suffering from diabetic neuropathy, alcohol abuse can exacerbate nerve damage. Alcohol interferes with the body's ability to regulate blood sugar levels, leading to increased nerve damage and worsening symptoms. Diabetic neuropathy patients should avoid alcohol consumption to prevent further deterioration of nerve function.

Chemotherapy-Induced Neuropathy:

Chemotherapy drugs used to treat cancer can also cause neuropathy. When combined with alcohol abuse, the risk of developing chemotherapy-induced neuropathy significantly increases. Alcohol can interact with chemotherapy drugs, leading to heightened toxicity and nerve damage. Patients undergoing chemotherapy should strictly avoid alcohol to minimize the risk of developing neuropathy.

Other Types of Neuropathy:

While alcohol abuse can exacerbate existing neuropathies, it can also contribute to the development of new ones. Small fiber neuropathy, idiopathic neuropathy, hereditary neuropathy, and neuropathy associated with HIV/AIDS or Lyme disease can all be influenced by alcohol consumption. Alcohol weakens the immune system, making individuals more susceptible to infections that can trigger or worsen these neuropathies.

Conclusion:

Alcohol abuse not only poses a threat to overall health but also significantly affects nerve function, leading to various types of neuropathy. Whether it is diabetic neuropathy, peripheral neuropathy, autonomic neuropathy, chemotherapy-induced neuropathy, small fiber neuropathy, idiopathic neuropathy, hereditary neuropathy, neuropathy associated with HIV/AIDS, neuropathy related to Lyme disease, or alcoholic neuropathy, the damaging effects of alcohol on nerve function are undeniable. It is crucial for individuals, especially those already suffering from neuropathy, to recognize the importance of abstaining from alcohol to preserve nerve health and prevent further complications. By making informed choices and seeking support when needed, individuals can take control of their health and mitigate the impact of alcohol abuse on nerve function.

Symptoms and Diagnosis of Alcoholic Neuropathy

Alcoholic neuropathy is a condition that affects individuals who have been long-term heavy drinkers. It is a type of peripheral neuropathy, which means it affects the nerves outside of the brain and spinal cord. Understanding the symptoms and getting an accurate diagnosis are crucial for managing this condition effectively.

The symptoms of alcoholic neuropathy can vary from person to person and often develop gradually over time. One of the most common symptoms is pain, which can range from mild to severe. Individuals may experience a burning or tingling sensation in their extremities, such as the hands and feet. This pain can be constant or intermittent and may worsen at night.

Another symptom of alcoholic neuropathy is muscle weakness. As the nerves become damaged, it can lead to a loss of muscle strength, making it difficult to perform everyday tasks. Some individuals may also experience muscle cramps or twitching.

Alcoholic neuropathy can also affect the autonomic nerves, which control involuntary bodily functions. This can lead to symptoms such as dizziness, lightheadedness, and problems with digestion, bladder control, and sexual function. Some individuals may also experience changes in blood pressure and heart rate.

Diagnosing alcoholic neuropathy involves a combination of medical history, physical examination, and diagnostic tests. It is crucial for individuals to be honest about their alcohol consumption habits, as this information helps healthcare professionals make an accurate diagnosis.

During the physical examination, a healthcare provider may check for muscle weakness, reflexes, and sensation in the affected areas. They may also order tests such as nerve conduction studies and electromyography to assess the function of the nerves and muscles.

In some cases, a nerve biopsy may be performed to examine a small sample of nerve tissue for signs of damage. Blood tests may also be conducted to rule out other possible causes of neuropathy, such as vitamin deficiencies or diabetes.

Once a diagnosis of alcoholic neuropathy is confirmed, it is essential to address the underlying cause by reducing or eliminating alcohol consumption. Treatment may also involve managing symptoms through medications, physical therapy, and lifestyle modifications.

In conclusion, recognizing the symptoms and obtaining an accurate diagnosis for alcoholic neuropathy is crucial for managing this condition effectively. By understanding the signs and seeking timely medical attention, individuals can take the necessary steps to improve their quality of life and prevent further nerve damage.

Rehabilitation and Lifestyle Changes for Alcoholic Neuropathy Patients

Alcoholic neuropathy is a condition that affects the nerves in individuals who have a history of heavy alcohol consumption. It can cause a range of symptoms such as tingling, numbness, muscle weakness, and pain in the extremities. However, with proper rehabilitation and lifestyle changes, patients can manage their symptoms and improve their quality of life.

One of the most important steps in rehabilitating alcoholic neuropathy patients is to stop drinking alcohol completely. Continued alcohol consumption can worsen the condition and increase the risk of developing further nerve damage. Quitting alcohol is not easy, but there are various support groups, counseling services, and treatment centers available to help individuals overcome their addiction.

In addition to quitting alcohol, lifestyle changes are crucial for managing alcoholic neuropathy. Regular exercise, such as walking or swimming, can help improve blood circulation and reduce neuropathic pain. Physical therapy might also be recommended to strengthen muscles and improve balance, as alcoholic neuropathy can often lead to muscle weakness and difficulty with coordination.

A healthy diet is another important aspect of managing alcoholic neuropathy. Consuming a balanced diet rich in vitamins and minerals, especially B vitamins, can help support nerve health and reduce symptoms. It is advisable to include foods like whole grains, fruits, vegetables, lean protein, and healthy fats in the diet. In some cases, a healthcare professional might also recommend vitamin supplements to ensure proper nutrient intake.

Managing pain is a significant concern for individuals with alcoholic neuropathy. Over-the-counter pain relievers or prescription medications may be prescribed to alleviate symptoms. However, it is essential to consult a healthcare professional before taking any medication, as they can advise on the appropriate dosage and potential side effects.

Furthermore, alternative therapies such as acupuncture, massage, and transcutaneous electrical nerve stimulation (TENS) have shown promise in managing neuropathic pain. These therapies can help reduce pain and improve overall well-being, but it is crucial to consult with a healthcare professional before starting any alternative treatment.

In conclusion, rehabilitation and lifestyle changes play a vital role in managing alcoholic neuropathy. By quitting alcohol, adopting a healthy lifestyle, and seeking appropriate medical care, individuals can alleviate their symptoms and improve their overall quality of life. It is essential to consult with healthcare professionals for personalized advice and support on the journey to recovery from alcoholic neuropathy.

Chapter 12: Living with Neuropathy: Coping Strategies and Support

Emotional and Psychological Impact of Neuropathy

Living with neuropathy can have a profound impact not only on the physical well-being of individuals but also on their emotional and psychological health. Understanding and managing the emotional and psychological aspects of neuropathy is crucial for those affected by this condition.

For individuals with diabetic neuropathy, the most common type of neuropathy, dealing with the physical symptoms such as tingling, numbness, and pain can be distressing. The chronic nature of the condition can lead to frustration, anger, and feelings of helplessness. It is not uncommon for individuals to experience anxiety and depression as a result of the constant pain and discomfort.

Peripheral neuropathy, which affects the nerves outside the brain and spinal cord, can also have a significant emotional impact. The loss of sensation and motor control in the limbs can lead to feelings of insecurity and fear. Individuals may worry about their ability to perform daily activities and fear falling or injuring themselves.

Autonomic neuropathy, which affects the nerves that control involuntary bodily functions, can disrupt the normal functioning of organs such as the heart, digestive system, and bladder. This can lead to anxiety, depression, and a sense of loss of control over one's own body.

Chemotherapy-induced neuropathy, a side effect of cancer treatment, can be emotionally and psychologically challenging. The physical symptoms, combined with the emotional strain of battling cancer, can lead to increased distress and anxiety.

Neuropathy associated with HIV/AIDS and Lyme disease can also take a toll on mental well-being. The uncertainty of living with a chronic illness and the physical limitations it imposes can lead to feelings of sadness, isolation, and anxiety about the future.

It is important for individuals with neuropathy to seek support and address their emotional and psychological well-being. Connecting with support groups, counseling, or therapy can provide a safe space to share experiences, learn coping strategies, and find emotional support.

In addition, adopting stress management techniques, practicing relaxation exercises, and engaging in activities that bring joy and fulfillment can help improve emotional well-being. Building a strong support network of friends, family, and healthcare professionals can also provide the necessary support and encouragement.

Understanding the emotional and psychological impact of neuropathy is crucial for both individuals and their loved ones. By addressing these aspects, individuals can work towards a more holistic approach to managing neuropathy and improving their overall quality of life.

Self-care and Lifestyle Modifications for Neuropathy Patients

Living with neuropathy can be challenging, but with the right self-care practices and lifestyle modifications, patients can effectively manage their condition and improve their quality of life. This subchapter focuses on providing practical tips and advice for individuals with various types of neuropathy, including diabetic neuropathy, peripheral neuropathy, autonomic neuropathy, chemotherapy-induced neuropathy, small fiber neuropathy, idiopathic neuropathy, hereditary neuropathy, neuropathy associated with HIV/AIDS, neuropathy related to Lyme disease, and alcoholic neuropathy.

1. Proper Foot Care: For individuals with diabetic neuropathy or peripheral neuropathy, taking care of the feet is crucial. Inspect your feet

daily for any signs of blisters, sores, or infections. Keep your feet clean and dry, and wear comfortable shoes that provide adequate support and protection.

2. Pain Management Techniques: Neuropathy often comes with chronic pain. Explore various pain management techniques, such as over-the-counter pain relievers, topical creams, heat or cold therapy, acupuncture, or nerve-stimulating devices. Consult with your healthcare provider to find the most suitable options for you.

3. Regular Exercise: Engaging in regular physical activity can help improve neuropathy symptoms and overall wellbeing. Opt for low-impact exercises like walking, swimming, or cycling to reduce stress on the nerves. Exercise also helps maintain a healthy weight, control blood sugar levels, and enhance circulation.

4. Balanced Diet: A healthy and well-balanced diet is essential for managing neuropathy. Focus on consuming nutrient-rich foods, including fruits, vegetables, whole grains, lean proteins, and healthy fats. Limit your intake of processed foods, sugary snacks, and alcohol, as they can worsen symptoms.

5. Stress Reduction Techniques: Stress can exacerbate neuropathy symptoms. Incorporate stress reduction techniques into your daily routine, such as deep breathing exercises, meditation, yoga, or engaging in hobbies that bring you joy. Consider seeking support from therapists or support groups to help cope with the emotional challenges of living with neuropathy.

6. Regular Check-ups: Regularly visit your healthcare provider to monitor your condition and make necessary adjustments to your treatment plan. They can also provide guidance on managing specific types of neuropathy and address any concerns or questions you may have.

Remember, self-care and lifestyle modifications are vital components of managing neuropathy. By implementing these practices into your daily routine, you can take control of your condition and lead a fulfilling life despite the challenges posed by neuropathy.

Note: It is important to consult with a healthcare professional for personalized advice and treatment options tailored to your specific neuropathy condition.

Seeking Support and Resources for Neuropathy Management

Living with neuropathy can be a challenging and overwhelming experience, but you don't have to face it alone. There are numerous support networks and resources available to help you better understand and manage your condition. Whether you are dealing with diabetic neuropathy, peripheral neuropathy, autonomic neuropathy, chemotherapy-induced neuropathy, small fiber neuropathy, idiopathic neuropathy, hereditary neuropathy, neuropathy associated with HIV/AIDS, neuropathy related to Lyme disease, or alcoholic neuropathy, this subchapter aims to guide you towards seeking the support and resources you need for effective neuropathy management.

Firstly, it is crucial to reach out to healthcare professionals who specialize in neuropathy. These experts, such as neurologists, endocrinologists, and pain management specialists, possess the knowledge and experience to diagnose and treat your specific type of neuropathy. They can provide you with tailored treatment plans and offer guidance on minimizing symptoms and preventing further nerve damage. Additionally, they may refer you to other healthcare providers who can offer complementary therapies such as physical therapy, occupational therapy, or acupuncture.

Support groups can also play a vital role in your journey. Connecting with others who are going through similar experiences can provide a sense of belonging and understanding. Sharing stories, tips, and coping strategies can be immensely helpful in managing both the physical and emotional aspects of neuropathy. Local hospitals, community centers, or online platforms can be excellent sources for finding support groups specific to your type of neuropathy.

Educating yourself about neuropathy is another essential step. There are numerous books, websites, and online forums dedicated to neuropathy education. These resources can provide you with valuable information on the causes, symptoms, treatments, and self-care techniques for neuropathy. Additionally, they may offer insights into the latest research and advancements in neuropathy management.

Financial and insurance assistance programs are available for those struggling to afford necessary treatments and medications. Organizations like the American Diabetes Association, Neuropathy Action Foundation, and Neuropathy Support Network can provide information on financial aid options, medication assistance programs, and insurance coverage.

In conclusion, seeking support and resources for neuropathy management is crucial for living a fulfilling life despite the challenges posed by this condition. By consulting healthcare professionals, joining support groups, educating yourself, and exploring financial assistance programs, you can arm yourself with the tools and knowledge needed to effectively manage your neuropathy and improve your overall well-being. Remember, you are not alone on this journey, and with the right support, you can regain control over your life.

Chapter 13: Future Directions in Neuropathy Research and Treatment

Advancements in Neuropathy Research

Neuropathy, a condition characterized by nerve damage, is a widespread problem that affects millions of people worldwide. While it can be associated with various underlying causes, such as diabetes, chemotherapy, HIV/AIDS, or alcoholism, the impact on individuals' lives is often similar. However, there is hope on the horizon as advancements in neuropathy research offer promising possibilities for understanding and managing this debilitating condition.

In recent years, researchers have made significant strides in unraveling the complexities of neuropathy. One area of focus has been diabetic neuropathy, a nerve disorder that commonly affects individuals with diabetes. Through extensive studies, scientists have gained a better understanding of the mechanisms behind nerve damage in diabetes and are exploring innovative treatment options. For instance, they are investigating the potential benefits of using stem cells to repair damaged nerves and developing new drugs specifically targeting the underlying causes of diabetic neuropathy.

Peripheral neuropathy, another common form of nerve damage, has also seen advancements in research. Scientists have been studying the role of genetics in peripheral neuropathy, which has led to a better understanding of hereditary neuropathies. This knowledge could pave the way for targeted therapies tailored to individuals' specific genetic makeup, improving treatment outcomes and quality of life.

Moreover, researchers have been delving into autonomic neuropathy, which affects the nerves regulating involuntary bodily functions like heart rate, digestion, and blood pressure. With advancements in imaging techniques, they have gained insights into the structural changes occurring within autonomic nerves, which may aid in developing more effective diagnostic tools and tailored treatment strategies.

Chemotherapy-induced neuropathy, a distressing side effect of cancer treatment, has also received considerable attention from the scientific community. Studies are underway to identify biomarkers that could predict the development of chemotherapy-induced neuropathy, allowing for early intervention and prevention. Additionally, researchers are exploring novel interventions, such as cryotherapy or electrical stimulation, to alleviate the symptoms and improve patients' quality of life during and after treatment.

The advancements in neuropathy research extend beyond specific conditions, as scientists are actively investigating idiopathic neuropathy, neuropathy associated with HIV/AIDS, neuropathy related to Lyme disease, and alcoholic neuropathy. By understanding the unique mechanisms and factors contributing to each type of neuropathy, researchers hope to develop tailored treatments that address the underlying causes and provide relief to those affected.

In conclusion, the field of neuropathy research is rapidly evolving, offering hope and promising advancements for individuals suffering from various forms of nerve damage. From diabetic neuropathy to peripheral neuropathy, autonomic neuropathy to chemotherapy-induced neuropathy, researchers are making significant strides towards understanding the mechanisms of nerve damage and developing targeted treatments. These advancements bring us closer to a future where neuropathy can be effectively managed, improving the lives of millions of people worldwide.

Promising Treatment Options on the Horizon

In recent years, significant strides have been made in the field of neuropathy research, giving hope to millions of individuals suffering from various forms of nerve damage. As we delve into the topic of promising treatment options on the horizon, it is important to understand that while some of these therapies are still in the experimental stages, they hold immense potential for the future management and potential reversal of neuropathy symptoms.

For individuals with diabetic neuropathy, a condition that affects a large number of people worldwide, research has shown promising results in certain medications and therapies. One such option is the use of neurotrophic factors, which are substances that promote the growth and survival of nerve cells. These factors have demonstrated the ability to repair damaged nerves and relieve diabetic neuropathy symptoms in clinical trials.

Additionally, advances in stem cell therapy have shown potential in the treatment of peripheral neuropathy, a condition that affects the nerves outside the central nervous system. Stem cells have the remarkable ability to differentiate into various types of cells, including nerve cells. By injecting these cells into damaged areas, researchers hope to stimulate nerve regeneration and restore functionality.

Another area of research that holds promise is autonomic neuropathy, which affects the nerves that control involuntary bodily functions. New treatment options focusing on the restoration of autonomic nerve function are being explored, including the use of vagus nerve stimulation and artificial intelligence-based techniques to regulate autonomic responses.

Chemotherapy-induced neuropathy, a common side effect of cancer treatment, has also attracted significant attention from researchers. Studies are underway to develop neuroprotective agents that can shield nerves from the toxic effects of chemotherapy drugs, thus reducing or preventing nerve damage.

Small fiber neuropathy, a condition characterized by damage to the small nerve fibers, has seen advancements in diagnostic techniques, enabling more accurate and targeted treatment approaches. With the help of skin biopsy, specialized nerve tests, and genetic testing, doctors can now identify the underlying causes of small fiber neuropathy and tailor treatment plans accordingly.

While the aforementioned treatment options offer hope to those with specific forms of neuropathy, it is important to note that research is also being conducted on a broader scale to address idiopathic neuropathy, hereditary neuropathy, neuropathy associated with HIV/AIDS, neuropathy related to Lyme disease, and alcoholic neuropathy. By understanding the mechanisms underlying these conditions, researchers aim to develop more effective treatments that can improve the quality of life for those affected.

As we move forward, it is crucial for the public to stay informed about the latest developments in neuropathy research. By fostering awareness and supporting ongoing studies, we can contribute to the advancement of treatment options and, ultimately, find a cure for this debilitating condition.

The Importance of Early Detection and Prevention in Neuropathy

Neuropathy, a condition characterized by damage to the nerves, can have a profound impact on an individual's quality of life. Whether it is caused by diabetes, chemotherapy, or other underlying factors, neuropathy can lead to a range of debilitating symptoms. However, the key to managing and mitigating the effects of neuropathy lies in early detection and prevention.

For individuals living with diabetic neuropathy, early detection is crucial in order to prevent further nerve damage. Diabetes is a leading cause of neuropathy, and as such, individuals with diabetes must be vigilant in monitoring their nerve health. Regular check-ups with healthcare professionals, including screenings for neuropathy, can help identify any signs of nerve damage before it progresses. By detecting neuropathy at an early stage, individuals can take proactive steps to prevent further damage and manage their symptoms effectively.

Similarly, individuals with peripheral neuropathy, autonomic neuropathy, chemotherapy-induced neuropathy, small fiber neuropathy, idiopathic neuropathy, hereditary neuropathy, or neuropathy associated with HIV/AIDS or Lyme disease, should also prioritize early detection. These various forms of neuropathy can have different causes and symptoms, but they all share the potential for long-term damage if left untreated.

Prevention is equally important in managing neuropathy. By adopting a proactive approach to nerve health, individuals can reduce their risk of developing neuropathy or mitigate its effects. This includes maintaining a healthy lifestyle, managing underlying conditions such as diabetes, monitoring medication side effects, and avoiding harmful substances like alcohol.

Early detection and prevention also play a crucial role in minimizing the impact of chemotherapy-induced neuropathy. Cancer treatments that involve chemotherapy can cause nerve damage, resulting in symptoms such as numbness, tingling, and pain. By identifying this type of neuropathy early on, healthcare professionals can adjust treatment plans and provide supportive care to alleviate symptoms and improve overall well-being.

In conclusion, early detection and prevention are essential in managing various forms of neuropathy. By being proactive in monitoring nerve health and taking steps to mitigate risk factors, individuals can minimize the impact of neuropathy and improve their overall quality of life. Regular screenings, lifestyle modifications, and effective management of underlying conditions are key strategies in the fight against neuropathy. By unveiling the importance of early detection and prevention, we can empower individuals to take control of their nerve health and live their lives to the fullest.

Chapter 14: Conclusion

Recap of Key Points

Understanding and managing neuropathy is crucial for individuals suffering from various forms of nerve damage. Whether you are dealing with diabetic neuropathy, peripheral neuropathy, autonomic neuropathy, chemotherapy-induced neuropathy, small fiber neuropathy, idiopathic neuropathy, hereditary neuropathy, neuropathy associated with HIV/AIDS, neuropathy related to Lyme disease, or alcoholic neuropathy, this recap of key points will provide you with essential information to help you navigate your condition.

1. Definition: Neuropathy refers to damage or dysfunction of the nerves, resulting in a range of symptoms such as pain, numbness, tingling, and weakness. It can affect different types of nerves, including sensory, motor, and autonomic nerves.

2. Causes: Neuropathy can be caused by various factors, including diabetes, certain medications, infections, autoimmune disorders, genetic mutations, and excessive alcohol consumption. Identifying the underlying cause is crucial for effective management.

3. Symptoms: Symptoms of neuropathy vary depending on the type and location of the nerve damage. Common symptoms include numbness or loss of sensation, tingling or burning sensations, muscle weakness, poor coordination, and changes in blood pressure or heart rate.

4. Diagnosis: Diagnosis often involves a thorough medical history review, physical examination, and specialized tests such as nerve conduction studies, electromyography, blood tests, and nerve biopsies. Accurate diagnosis is essential to determine the appropriate treatment plan.

5. Treatment Options: Treatment for neuropathy focuses on managing symptoms, preventing further nerve damage, and addressing the underlying cause when possible. This may involve a combination of medication, physical therapy, lifestyle modifications, pain management techniques, and alternative therapies like acupuncture or nerve stimulation.

6. Self-care Strategies: Self-care plays a vital role in managing neuropathy. It includes maintaining good blood sugar control for diabetic neuropathy patients, regular exercise to improve circulation, proper foot care, quitting smoking, and adopting a healthy lifestyle that promotes nerve health.

7. Support and Resources: Living with neuropathy can be challenging, both physically and emotionally. Seek support from healthcare professionals, support groups, and online communities that specialize in neuropathy. They can provide valuable information, resources, and emotional support.

Remember, managing neuropathy requires a multidisciplinary approach, involving healthcare professionals, self-care, and support systems. By understanding the key points discussed above, you can take control of your condition and improve your quality of life.

Empowering Individuals with Neuropathy

Living with neuropathy can be a challenging and overwhelming experience. Whether you are dealing with diabetic neuropathy, peripheral neuropathy, autonomic neuropathy, chemotherapy-induced neuropathy, small fiber neuropathy, idiopathic neuropathy, hereditary neuropathy, neuropathy associated with HIV/AIDS, neuropathy related to Lyme disease, or alcoholic neuropathy, it is important to understand that you are not alone. This subchapter aims to empower individuals with neuropathy by providing valuable information and strategies for managing and coping with this condition.

First and foremost, education is key. Understanding the causes, symptoms, and progression of neuropathy can help individuals make informed decisions about their treatment and lifestyle choices. This book, "Neuropathy Unveiled: Understanding and Managing Diabetic Nerve Damage," serves as a comprehensive guide to neuropathy, providing clear explanations and insights into the various types of neuropathy and their impact on daily life.

One of the most crucial aspects of managing neuropathy is adopting a proactive approach to self-care. This includes paying close attention to one's overall health and making lifestyle changes that can alleviate symptoms and prevent further nerve damage. Simple modifications such as maintaining a healthy diet, exercising regularly, managing stress levels, and avoiding harmful substances like alcohol and tobacco can make a significant difference in managing neuropathy.

Additionally, seeking medical guidance and support is essential. Consulting with healthcare professionals who specialize in neuropathy can provide valuable insights and personalized treatment plans. They can offer a range of treatment options, including medications, physical therapy, occupational therapy, and alternative therapies such as acupuncture or nerve stimulation techniques.

Support groups and online communities can also play a vital role in empowering individuals with neuropathy. Sharing experiences, exchanging tips and advice, and connecting with others who are facing similar challenges can provide a sense of validation and support. These communities can offer a safe space for individuals to express their concerns, ask questions, and learn from others' experiences.

Finally, it is crucial to remember that living with neuropathy does not define who you are as an individual. Despite the physical and emotional challenges, there are still plenty of opportunities to lead a fulfilling life. Exploring new hobbies, setting realistic goals, and maintaining social connections with loved ones can help individuals regain a sense of purpose and happiness.

In conclusion, this subchapter aims to empower individuals with neuropathy by providing them with the knowledge, resources, and support they need to effectively manage their condition. By understanding the various types of neuropathy and implementing self-care strategies, seeking medical guidance, connecting with support networks, and embracing a positive mindset, individuals can regain control over their lives and live to their fullest potential.

Encouragement for a Better Quality of Life

Living with neuropathy can be challenging, but it doesn't have to define your life. With the right mindset and proactive approach, you can improve your quality of life and find ways to manage the symptoms associated with diabetic nerve damage and other types of neuropathy. Here are some encouraging tips and strategies to help you navigate this journey towards a better quality of life.

1. Education and Awareness: Knowledge is power when it comes to managing neuropathy. Take the time to understand your specific condition, its causes, symptoms, and available treatment options. By being well-informed, you can actively participate in your own care and make informed decisions.

2. Healthy Lifestyle Choices: A healthy lifestyle plays a vital role in managing neuropathy. Focus on maintaining a balanced diet, rich in essential nutrients, and low in sugar. Regular exercise, such as walking or swimming, can help improve circulation and alleviate symptoms. Avoid

smoking and excessive alcohol consumption as they can worsen neuropathy symptoms.

3. Pain Management Techniques: Chronic pain is a common symptom of neuropathy, but it doesn't have to control your life. Explore various pain management techniques such as physical therapy, acupuncture, meditation, or relaxation exercises. Work closely with your healthcare provider to find the right combination of treatments that work for you.

4. Support Networks: Seek support from others who understand what you're going through. Join local or online support groups, where you can share experiences, gain valuable insights, and find emotional support. Remember, you're not alone on this journey, and connecting with others can make a significant difference.

5. Self-Care and Stress Reduction: Prioritize self-care activities that promote relaxation and reduce stress levels. Engage in hobbies you enjoy, practice mindfulness or deep breathing exercises, express yourself through art or music, or pamper yourself with a soothing bath or massage. By managing stress, you can minimize the impact it has on your neuropathy symptoms.

6. Regular Check-ups: Regular visits to your healthcare provider are crucial for monitoring your condition and adjusting treatment plans when necessary. Stay proactive in managing your health by scheduling routine check-ups, following prescribed medications, and staying informed about the latest advancements in neuropathy treatments.

Remember, neuropathy may present unique challenges, but it doesn't have to limit your potential for a fulfilling life. By adopting these strategies and maintaining a positive mindset, you can take control of your neuropathy and work towards a better quality of life. Stay hopeful, stay determined, and seek the support you need to thrive despite the challenges.

Appendix: Resources and References

In this appendix, we have compiled a list of valuable resources and references for individuals seeking further information and support related to neuropathy. Whether you are living with diabetic neuropathy, peripheral neuropathy, autonomic neuropathy, chemotherapy-induced neuropathy, small fiber neuropathy, idiopathic neuropathy, hereditary neuropathy, neuropathy associated with HIV/AIDS, neuropathy related to Lyme disease, or alcoholic neuropathy, these resources can provide you with knowledge, guidance, and assistance in managing your condition effectively.

National Institute of Diabetes and Digestive and Kidney Diseases (NIDDK): The NIDDK offers a comprehensive website dedicated to diabetes and its complications, including diabetic neuropathy. You can find information on symptoms, treatment options, and self-care strategies.

The Neuropathy Association: This nonprofit organization focuses on providing support, education, and resources to individuals living with all types of neuropathy. Their website offers a wealth of information on various neuropathies, treatment options, and access to support groups.

American Diabetes Association (ADA): The ADA is a trusted source for information on diabetes and its related complications. Their website provides comprehensive resources on diabetic neuropathy, including prevention, management, and lifestyle tips.

Foundation for Peripheral Neuropathy: This organization is dedicated to increasing awareness and understanding of peripheral neuropathy. Their website offers educational resources, research updates, and a patient forum for individuals seeking support and guidance.

Neuropathy Support Network: This online community serves as a platform for patients, caregivers, and healthcare professionals to connect and share experiences. The website provides information on various neuropathies and offers support through forums, webinars, and educational materials.

Mayo Clinic: The Mayo Clinic's website provides reliable information on a wide range of health topics, including neuropathy. You can find detailed articles on symptoms, causes, diagnosis, and treatment options for different types of neuropathies.

National Organization for Rare Disorders (NORD): NORD offers resources and support for individuals living with rare neuropathies, including hereditary and idiopathic neuropathies. Their website provides information on specific conditions, treatment options, and patient advocacy.

Centers for Disease Control and Prevention (CDC): The CDC offers information on neuropathy associated with HIV/AIDS and Lyme disease. Their website provides guidance on prevention, symptoms, and treatment options for these specific types of neuropathies.

Remember, this list is not exhaustive, and there are many other valuable resources available. It is always advisable to consult with healthcare professionals and specialists to ensure accurate diagnosis and personalized treatment plans.

By utilizing these resources and references, you can empower yourself with knowledge and gain a better understanding of neuropathy. Remember, you are not alone in your journey towards managing and overcoming neuropathy, and there is support available to help you lead a fulfilling life.